Ketogenic

Recipes

Effective Low-Carb Recipes To Balance Hormones And Effortlessly Reach Your Weight Loss Goal.

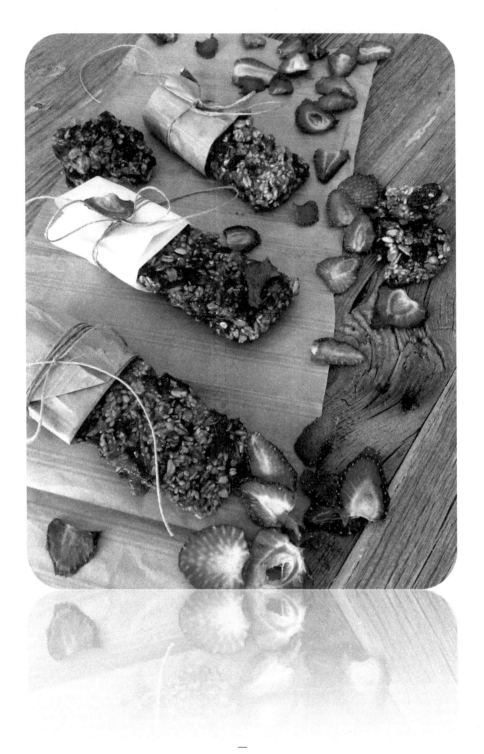

Introduction

Do you want to make a change in your life? Do you want to become a healthier person who can enjoy a new and improved life? Then, you are definitely in the right place. You are about to discover a wonderful and very healthy diet that has changed millions of lives. We are talking about the Ketogenic diet, a lifestyle that will mesmerize you and that will make you a new person in no time.

So, let's sit back, relax and find out more about the Ketogenic diet. A keto diet is a low carb one. This is the first and one of the most important things you should now. During such a diet, your body makes ketones in your liver and these are used as energy.

Your body will produce less insulin and glucose and a state of ketosis is induced. Ketosis is a natural process that appears when our food intake is lower than usual. The body will soon adapt to this state and therefore you will be able to lose weight in no time but you will also become healthier and your physical and mental performances will improve.

Your blood sugar levels will improve and you won't be predisposed to diabetes. Also, epilepsy and heart diseases can be prevented if you are on a Ketogenic diet. Your cholesterol will improve and you will feel amazing in no time. How does that sound?

A Ketogenic diet is simple and easy to follow as long as you follow some simple rules. You don't need to make huge changes but there are some things you should know.

So, here goes!

If you are on a Ketogenic diet you can't eat:

Grains like corn, cereals, rice, etc
Fruits like bananas
Sugar
Dry beans
Honey
Potatoes
Yams

If you are on a Ketogenic diet you can eat:

Greens like spinach, green beans, kale, bok choy, etc
Meat like poultry, fish, pork, lamb, beef, etc
Eggs
Above ground veggies like cauliflower or broccoli,
napa cabbage or
regular cabbage
Nuts and seeds
Cheese
Ghee or butter
Avocados and all kind of berries
Sweeteners like erythritol, splenda, stevia and others
that contain
only a few carbs
Coconut oil
Avocado oil
Olive oil

The list of foods you are allowed to eat during a keto
diet is permissive and rich as you can see for yourself.

—

So, we think it should be pretty easy for you to start such a diet.
If you've made this choice already, then, it's time you checked our amazing keto recipe collection.

You will discover 30 of the best ketogenic breakfast recipes, all with pictures, and you will soon he will be able to prepare each of these recipes.

Now let's start our magical culinary journey!

Ketogenic lifestyle...here we come!

Enjoy!

Delicious Poached Eggs

If you are on a Ketogenic diet, then this recipe is perfect for breakfast!

Preparation time: 10 minutes Cooking time: 35 minutes
Servings: 4

Ingredients:

3 garlic cloves, minced
1 tablespoon ghee
1 white onion, chopped
1 Serrano pepper, chopped
Salt and black pepper to the taste
1 red bell pepper, chopped
3 tomatoes, chopped
1 teaspoon paprika
1 teaspoon cumin
¼ teaspoon chili powder
1 tablespoon cilantro, chopped
6 eggs

Directions:

1. Heat up a pan with the ghee over medium heat, add onion, stir and cook for 10 minutes.
2. Add Serrano pepper and garlic, stir and cook for 1 minute.
3. Add red bell pepper, stir and cook for 10 minutes.
4. Add tomatoes, salt, pepper, chili powder, cumin and paprika, stir and cook for 10 minutes.
5. Crack eggs into the pan, season them with salt and pepper, cover pan and cook for 6 minutes more.
6. Sprinkle cilantro at the end and serve.
Enjoy!

Nutrition: calories 300, fat 12, fiber 3.4, carbs 22, protein 14

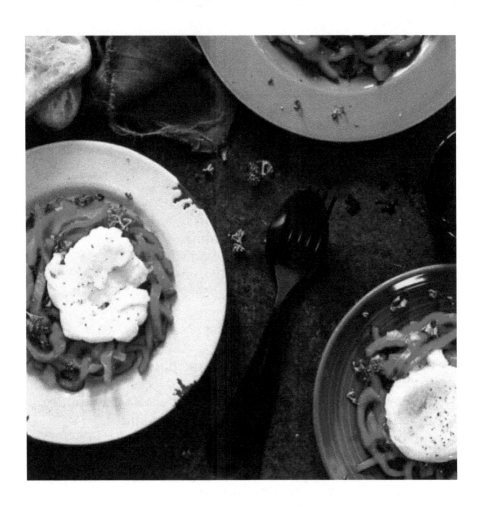

Delicious Breakfast Bowl

You will feel full of energy all day with this keto breakfast!

Preparation time: 10 minutes Cooking time: 20 minutes
Servings: 1

Ingredients:

4 ounces beef, ground
1 yellow onion, chopped
8 mushrooms, sliced
Salt and black pepper to the taste
2 eggs, whisked
1 tablespoon coconut oil
½ teaspoon smoked paprika
1 avocado, pitted, peeled and chopped
12 black olives, pitted and sliced

Directions:

1. Heat up a pan with the coconut oil over medium heat, add onions, mushrooms, salt and pepper, stir and cook for 5 minutes.
2. Add beef and paprika, stir, cook for 10 minutes and transfer to a bowl.
3. Heat up the pan again over medium heat, add eggs, some salt and pepper and scramble them.
4. Return beef mix to pan and stir.
5. Add avocado and olives, stir and cook for 1 minute.
6. Transfer to a bowl and serve.
Enjoy!

Nutrition: calories 600, fat 23, fiber 8, carbs 22, protein 43

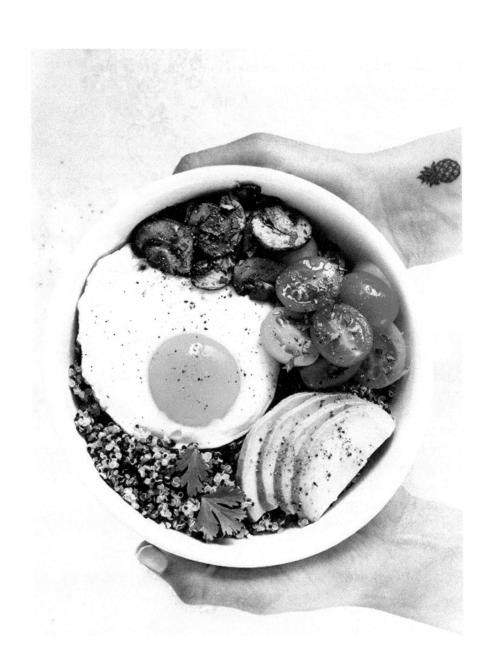

Delicious Eggs And Sausages

Try a different keto breakfast each day! Try this one!

Preparation time: 10 minutes Cooking time: 35 minutes
Servings: 6

Ingredients:

5 tablespoons ghee
12 eggs
Salt and black pepper to the taste
1-ounce spinach, torn
12 ham slices
2 sausages, chopped
1 yellow onion, chopped
1 red bell pepper, chopped

Directions:

1. Heat up a pan with 1 tablespoon ghee over medium heat, add sausages and onion, stir and cook for 5 minutes.
2. Add bell pepper, salt and pepper, stir and cook for 3 minutes more and transfer to a bowl.
3. Melt the rest of the ghee and divide into 12 cupcake molds.
4. Add a slice of ham in each cupcake mold, divide spinach in each and then the sausage mix.
5. Crack an egg on top, introduce everything in the oven and bake at 425 degrees F for 20 minutes.
6. Leave your keto cupcakes to cool down a bit before serving. Enjoy!

Nutrition: calories 440, fat 32, fiber 0, carbs 12, protein 22

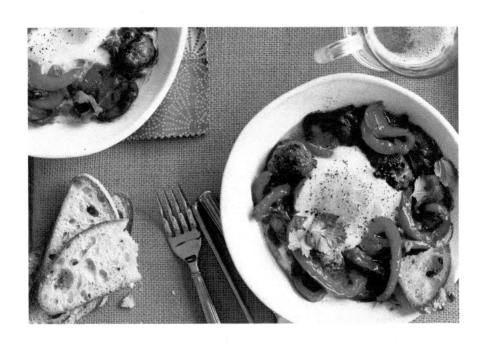

Scrambled Eggs

They taste delicious!

Preparation time: 10 minutes Cooking time: 10 minutes
Servings: 1

Ingredients:

4 bell mushrooms, chopped
3 eggs, whisked
Salt and black pepper to the taste
2 ham slices, chopped
¼ cup red bell pepper, chopped
½ cup spinach, chopped
1 tablespoon coconut oil

Directions:

1. Heat up a pan with half of the oil over medium heat, add mushrooms, spinach, ham and bell pepper, stir and cook for 4 minutes.
2. Heat up another pan with the rest of the oil over medium heat, add eggs and scramble them.
3. Add veggies and ham, salt and pepper, stir, cook for 1 minute and serve.
Enjoy!

Nutrition: calories 350, fat 23, fiber 1, carbs 5, protein 22

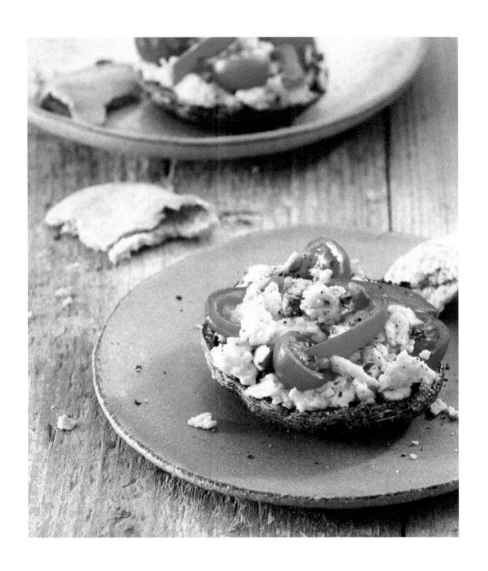

Delicious Frittata

Try a keto frittata today! It's so tasty!

Preparation time: 10 minutes Cooking time: 1 hour Servings: 4

Ingredients:

9 ounces spinach
12 eggs
1-ounce pepperoni
1 teaspoon garlic, minced
Salt and black pepper to the taste
5 ounces mozzarella, shredded
½ cup parmesan, grated
½ cup ricotta cheese
4 tablespoons olive oil
A pinch of nutmeg

Directions:

1. Squeeze liquid from spinach and put in a bowl.
2. In another bowl, mix eggs with salt, pepper, nutmeg and garlic and whisk well.
3. Add spinach, parmesan and ricotta and whisk well again.
4. Pour this into a pan, sprinkle mozzarella and pepperoni on top, introduce in the oven and bake at 375 degrees F for 45 minutes.
5. Leave frittata to cool down for a few minutes before serving it.
Enjoy!

Nutrition: calories 298, fat 2, fiber 1, carbs 6, protein 18

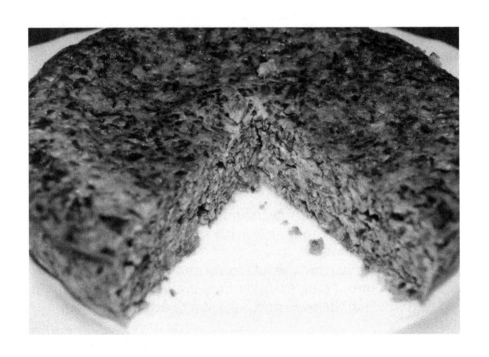

Smoked Salmon Breakfast

It will surprise you with its taste!

Preparation time: 10 minutes Cooking time: 10 minutes
Servings: 3

Ingredients:

4 eggs, whisked
½ teaspoon avocado oil
4 ounces smoked salmon, chopped
For the sauce:
1 cup coconut milk
½ cup cashews, soaked, drained
¼ cup green onions, chopped
1 teaspoon garlic powder
Salt and black pepper to the taste
1 tablespoon lemon juice

Directions:

1. In your blender, mix cashews with coconut milk, garlic powder and lemon juice and blend well.
2. Add salt, pepper and green onions, blend again well, transfer to a bowl and keep in the fridge for now.
3. Heat up a pan with the oil over medium-low heat, add eggs, whisk a bit and cook until they are almost done
4. Introduce in your preheated broiler and cook until eggs set.
5. Divide eggs on plates, top with smoked salmon and serve with the green onion sauce on top.
Enjoy!

Nutrition: calories 200, fat 10, fiber 2, carbs 11, protein 15

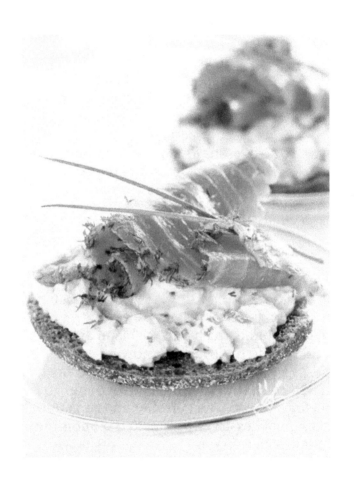

Feta And Asparagus Delight

These elements combine very well!

Preparation time: 10 minutes Cooking time: 25 minutes
Servings: 2

Ingredients:

12 asparagus spears
1 tablespoon olive oil
2 green onions, chopped
1 garlic clove, minced
6 eggs
Salt and black pepper to the taste
½ cup feta cheese

Directions:

1. Heat up a pan with some water over medium heat, add asparagus, cook for 8 minutes, drain well, chop 2 spears and reserve the rest.
2. Heat up a pan with the oil over medium heat, add garlic, chopped asparagus and onions, stir and cook for 5 minutes.
3. Add eggs, salt and pepper, stir, cover and cook for 5 minutes.
4. Arrange the whole asparagus on top of your frittata, sprinkle cheese, introduce in the oven at 350 degrees F and bake for 9 minutes.
5. Divide between plates and serve.
Enjoy!

Nutrition: calories 340, fat 12, fiber 3, carbs 8, protein 26

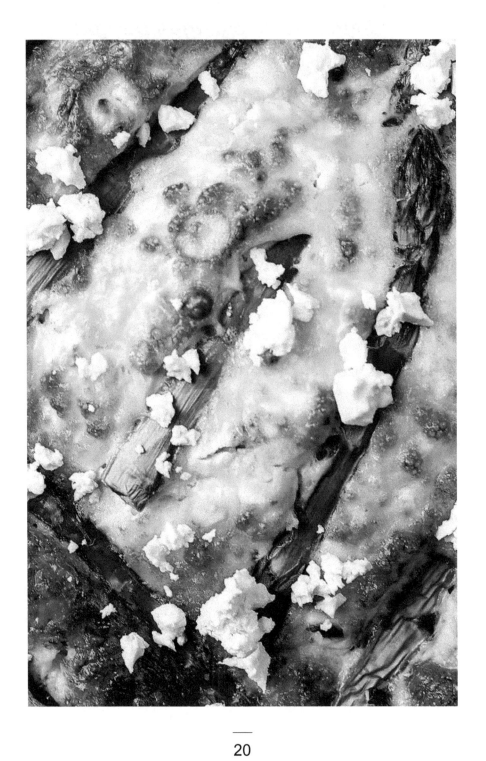

Special Breakfast Eggs

This is truly the best keto eggs recipe you can ever try!

Preparation time: 10 minutes Cooking time: 4 minutes
Servings: 12

Ingredients:

4 tea bags
4 tablespoons salt
12 eggs
2 tablespoons cinnamon
6-star anise
1 teaspoon black pepper
1 tablespoons peppercorns
8 cups water
1 cup tamari sauce

Directions:

1. Put water in a pot, add eggs, bring them to a boil over medium heat and cook until they are hard boiled.
2. Cool them down and crack them without peeling.
3. In a large pot, mix water with tea bags, salt, pepper, peppercorns, cinnamon, star anise and tamari sauce.
4. Add cracked eggs, cover pot, bring to a simmer over low heat and cook for 30 minutes.
5. Discard tea bags and cook eggs for 3 hours and 30 minutes.
6. Leave eggs to cool down, peel and serve them for breakfast. Enjoy!

Nutrition: calories 90, fat 6, fiber 0, carbs 0, protein 7

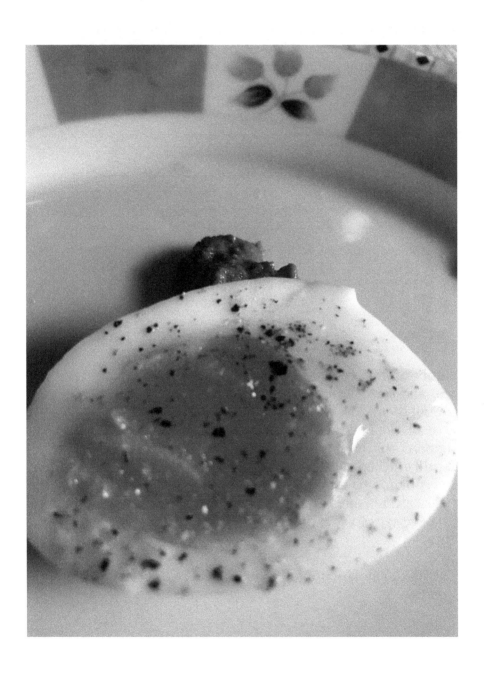

Eggs Baked In Avocados

They are so delicious and they look great too!

Preparation time: 10 minutes Cooking time: 20 minutes
Servings: 4

Ingredients:

2 avocados, cut in halves and pitted
4 eggs
Salt and black pepper to the taste
1 tablespoon chives, chopped

Directions:

1. Scoop some flesh from the avocado halves and arrange them in a baking dish.
2. Crack an egg in each avocado, season with salt and pepper, introduce them in the oven at 425 degrees F and bake for 20 minutes.
3. Sprinkle chives at the end and serve for breakfast!
Enjoy!

Nutrition: calories 400, fat 34, fiber 13, carbs 13, protein 15

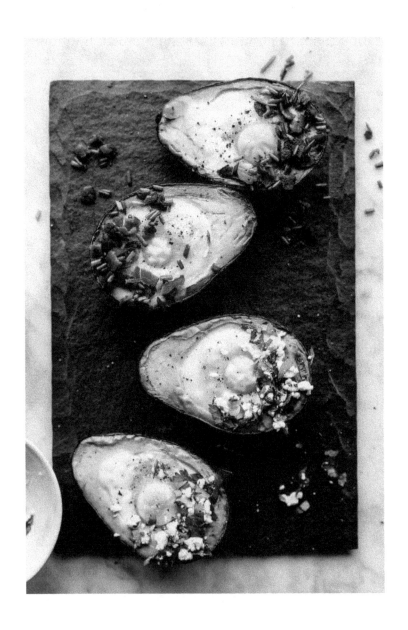

Shrimp And Bacon Breakfast

This is a perfect breakfast idea!

Preparation time: 10 minutes Cooking time: 15 minutes
Servings: 4

Ingredients:

1 cup mushrooms, sliced
4 bacon slices, chopped
4 ounces smoked salmon, chopped
4 ounces shrimp, deveined
Salt and black pepper to the taste
½ cup coconut cream

Directions:

1. Heat up a pan over medium heat, add bacon, stir and cook for 5 minutes.
2. Add mushrooms, stir and cook for 5 minutes more.
3. Add salmon, stir and cook for 3 minutes.
4. Add shrimp and cook for 2 minutes.
5. Add salt, pepper and coconut cream, stir, cook for 1 minute, take off heat and divide between plates.
Enjoy!

Nutrition: calories 340, fat 23, fiber 1, carbs 4, protein 17

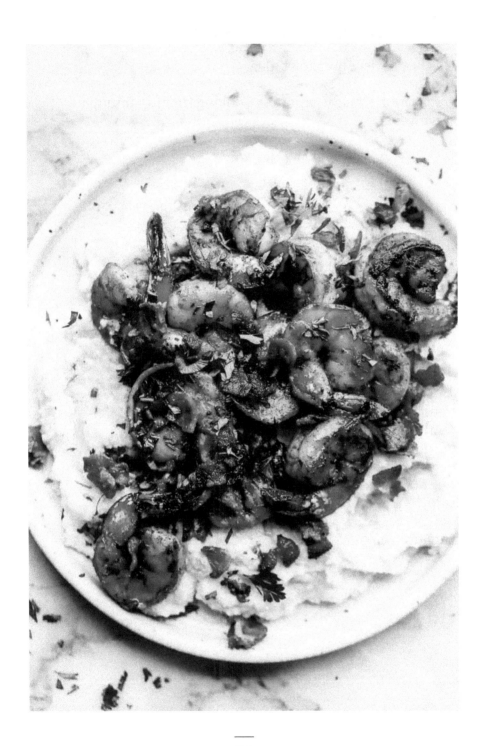

Delicious Mexican Breakfast

Try a Ketogenic Mexican breakfast today!

Preparation time: 10 minutes Cooking time: 30 minutes
Servings: 8

Ingredients:

½ cup enchilada sauce
1 pound pork, ground
1 pound chorizo, chopped
Salt and black pepper to the taste
8 eggs
1 tomato, chopped
3 tablespoons ghee
½ cup red onion, chopped
1 avocado, pitted, peeled and chopped

Directions:

1. In a bowl, mix pork with chorizo, stir and spread on a lined baking form.
2. Spread enchilada sauce on top, introduce in the oven at 350 degrees F and bake for 20 minutes.
3. Heat up a pan with the ghee over medium heat, add eggs and scramble them well.
4. Take pork mix out of the oven and spread scrambled eggs over them.
5. Sprinkle salt, pepper, tomato, onion and avocado, divide between plates and serve.
Enjoy!

Nutrition: calories 400, fat 32, fiber 4, carbs 7, protein 25

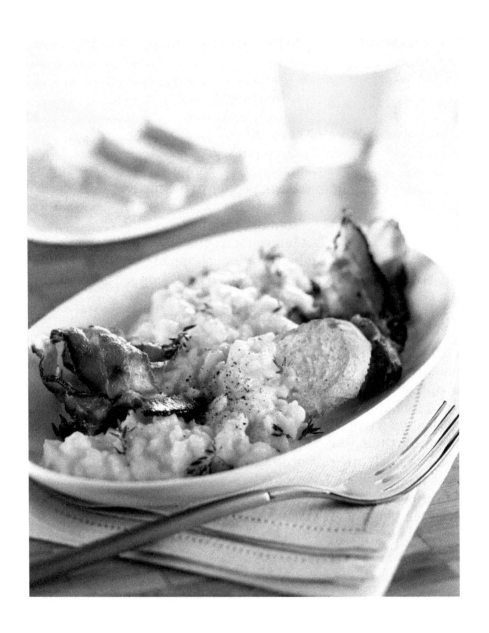

Delicious Breakfast Pie

Pay attention and learn how to make this great breakfast in no time!

Preparation time: 10 minutes Cooking time: 45 minutes
Servings: 8

Ingredients:

½ onion, chopped
1 pie crust
½ red bell pepper, chopped
¾ pound beef, ground
Salt and black pepper to the taste
3 tablespoons taco seasoning
A handful cilantro, chopped
8 eggs
1 teaspoon coconut oil
1 teaspoon baking soda
Mango salsa for serving

Directions:

1. Heat up a pan with the oil over medium heat, add beef, cook until it browns and mixes with salt, pepper and taco seasoning.
2. Stir again, transfer to a bowl and leave aside for now.
3. Heat up the pan again over medium heat with cooking juices from the meat, add onion and bell pepper, stir and cook for 4 minutes.
4. Add eggs, baking soda and some salt and stir well.
5. Add cilantro, stir again and take off heat.
6. Spread beef mix in pie crust, add veggies mix and spread over meat, introduce in the oven at 350 degrees F and bake for 45 minutes.
7. Leave the pie to cool down a bit, slice, divide between plates and serve with mango salsa on top.
Enjoy!

Nutrition: calories 198, fat 11, fiber 1, carbs 12, protein 12

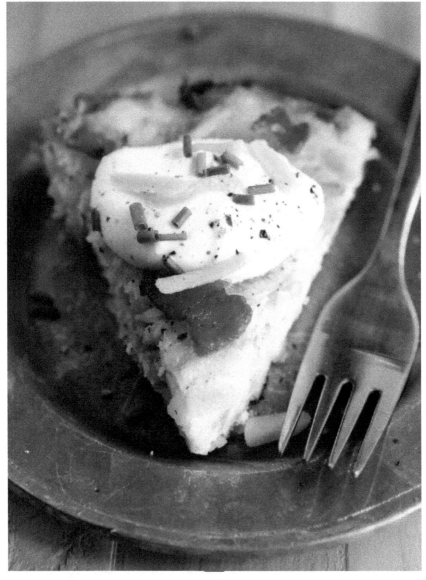

Breakfast Stir Fry

We recommend you try this keto breakfast as soon as possible!

Preparation time: 10 minutes Cooking time: 30 minutes
Servings: 2

Ingredients:

½ pounds beef meat, minced
2 teaspoons red chili flakes
1 tablespoon tamari sauce
2 bell peppers, chopped
1 teaspoon chili powder
1 tablespoon coconut oil
Salt and black pepper to the taste
For the bok choy:
6 bunches bok choy, trimmed and chopped
1 teaspoon ginger, grated
Salt to the taste
1 tablespoon coconut oil
For the eggs:
1 tablespoon coconut oil
2 eggs

Directions:

1. Heat up a pan with 1 tablespoon coconut oil over medium high heat, add beef and bell peppers, stir and cook for 10 minutes.
2. Add salt, pepper, tamari sauce, chili flakes and chili powder, stir, cook for 4 minutes more and take off heat.
3. Heat up another pan with 1 tablespoon oil over medium heat, add bok choy, stir and cook for 3 minutes.
4. Add salt and ginger, stir, cook for 2 minutes more and take off heat.
5. Heat up the third pan with 1 tablespoon oil over medium heat, crack eggs and fry them.
6. Divide beef and bell peppers mix into 2 bowls.

7. Divide bok choy and top with eggs.
Enjoy!

Nutrition: calories 248, fat 14, fiber 4, carbs 10, protein 14

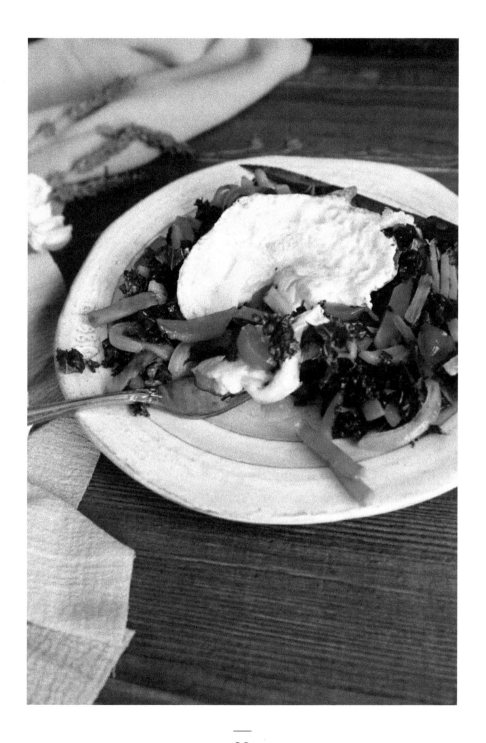

Delicious Breakfast Skillet

It's going to be so tasty!

Preparation time: 10 minutes Cooking time: 30 minutes
Servings: 4

Ingredients:

8 ounces mushrooms, chopped
Salt and black pepper to the taste
1 pound pork, minced
1 tablespoon coconut oil
½ teaspoon garlic powder
½ teaspoon basil, dried
2 tablespoons Dijon mustard
2 zucchinis, chopped

Directions:

1. Heat up a pan with the oil over medium high heat, add mushrooms, stir and cook for 4 minutes.
2. Add zucchinis, salt and pepper, stir and cook for 4 minutes more.
3. Add pork, garlic powder, basil, more salt and pepper, stir and cook until meat is done.
4. Add mustard, stir, cook for 3 minutes more, divide into bowls and serve.
Enjoy!

Nutrition: calories 240, fat 15, fiber 2, carbs 9, protein 17

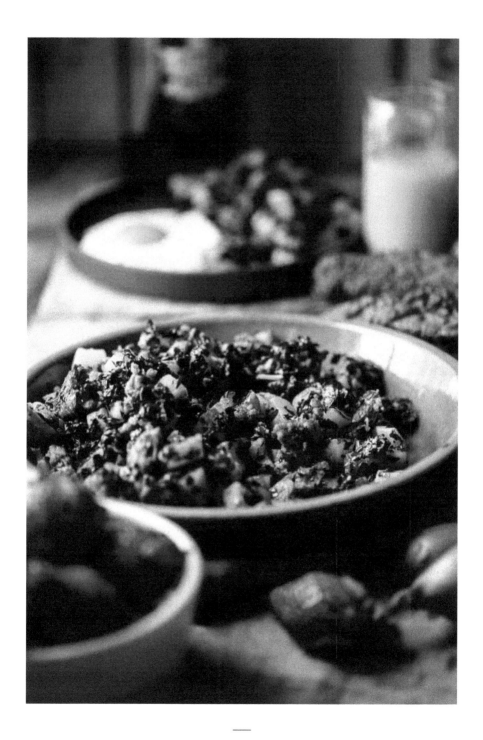

Breakfast Casserole

You've got to try this!

Preparation time: 10 minutes Cooking time: 40 minutes
Servings: 4

Ingredients:

10 eggs
1 pound pork sausage, chopped
1 yellow onion, chopped
3 cups spinach, torn
Salt and black pepper to the taste
3 tablespoons avocado oil

Directions:

1. Heat up a pan with 1 tablespoon oil over medium heat, add sausage, stir and brown it for 4 minutes.
2. Add onion, stir and cook for 3 minutes more.
3. Add spinach, stir and cook for 1 minute.
4. Grease a baking dish with the rest of the oil and spread sausage mix.
5. Whisk eggs and add them to sausage mix.
6. Stir gently, introduce in the oven at 350 degrees F and bake for 30 minutes.
7. Leave casserole to cool down for a few minutes before serving it for breakfast.
Enjoy!

Nutrition: calories 345, fat 12, fiber 1, carbs 8, protein 22

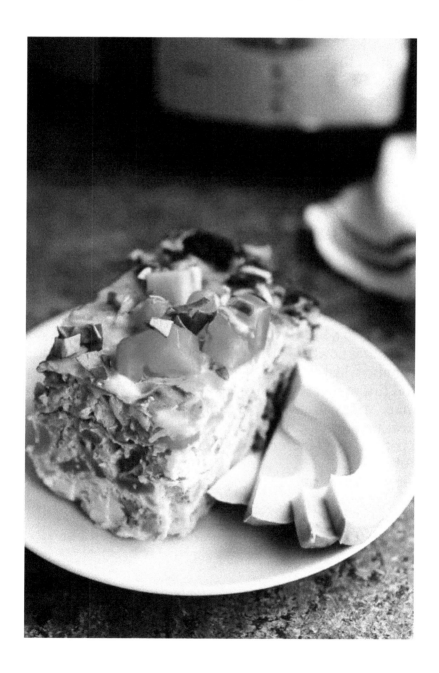

Incredible Breakfast Patties

This is incredibly tasty and easy to make for breakfast!

Preparation time: 10 minutes Cooking time: 10 minutes
Servings: 4

Ingredients:

1 pound pork meat, minced
Salt and black pepper to the taste
¼ teaspoon thyme, dried
½ teaspoon sage, dried
¼ teaspoon ginger, dried
3 tablespoon cold water
1 tablespoon coconut oil

Directions:

1. Put meat in a bowl.
2. In another bowl, mix water with salt, pepper, sage, thyme and ginger and whisk well.
3. Add this to meat and stir very well.
4. Shape your patties and place them on a working surface.
5. Heat up a pan with the coconut oil over medium high heat, add patties, fry them for 5 minutes, flip and cook them for 3 minutes more.
6. Serve them warm.
Enjoy!

Nutrition: calories 320, fat 13, fiber 2, carbs 10, protein 12

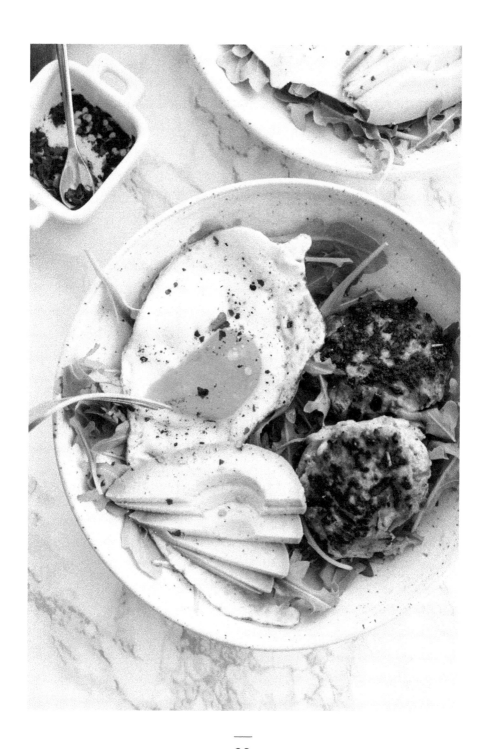

Delicious Sausage Quiche

It's so amazing! You must make it for breakfast tomorrow!

Preparation time: 10 minutes Cooking time: 40 minutes
Servings: 6

Ingredients:

12 ounces pork sausage, chopped
Salt and black pepper to the taste
2 teaspoons whipping cream
2 tablespoons parsley, chopped
10 mixed cherry tomatoes, halved
6 eggs
2 tablespoons parmesan, grated
5 eggplant slices

Directions:

1. Spread sausage pieces on the bottom of a baking dish.
2. Layer eggplant slices on top.
3. Add cherry tomatoes.
4. In a bowl, mix eggs with salt, pepper, cream and parmesan and whisk well.
5. Pour this into the baking dish, introduce in the oven at 375 degrees F and bake for 40 minutes.
6. Serve right away.
Enjoy!

Nutrition: calories 340, fat 28, fiber 3, carbs 3, protein 17

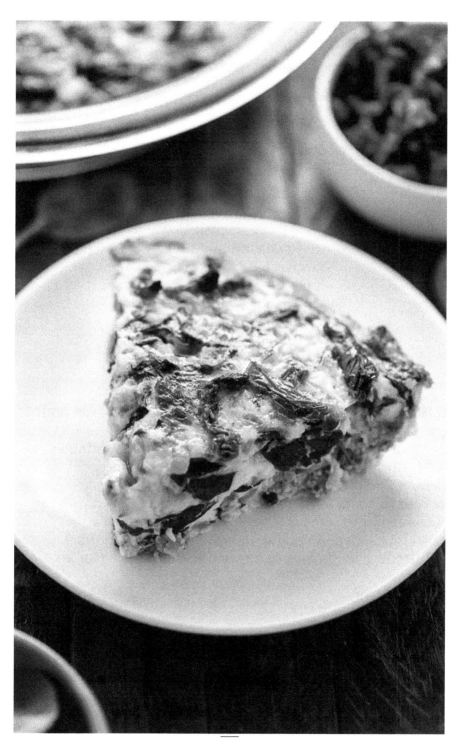

Special Breakfast Dish

This is a Ketogenic breakfast worth trying!

Preparation time: 10 minutes Cooking time: 40 minutes
Servings: 6

Ingredients:

1 pound sausage, chopped
1 leek, chopped
8 eggs, whisked
¼ cup coconut milk
6 asparagus stalks, chopped
1 tablespoon dill, chopped
Salt and black pepper to the taste
¼ teaspoon garlic powder
1 tablespoon coconut oil, melted

Directions:

1. Heat up a pan over medium heat, add sausage pieces and brown them for a few minutes.
2. Add asparagus and leek, stir and cook for a few minutes.
3. Meanwhile, in a bowl, mix eggs with salt, pepper, dill, garlic powder and coconut milk and whisk well.
4. Pour this into a baking dish which you've greased with the coconut oil.
5. Add sausage and veggies on top and whisk everything.
6. Introduce in the oven at 325 degrees F and bake for 40 minutes.
7. Serve warm.
Enjoy!

Nutrition: calories 340, fat 12, fiber 3, carbs 8, protein 23

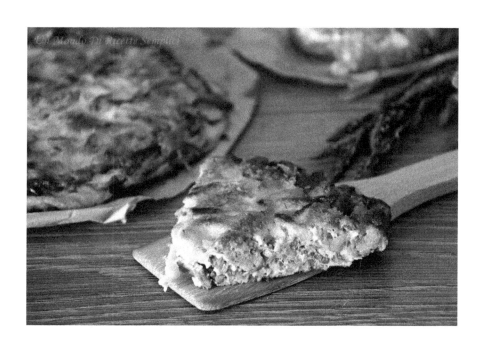

Chorizo And Cauliflower Breakfast

You don't need to be an expert cook to make a great breakfast! Try this next recipe and enjoy!

Preparation time: 10 minutes Cooking time: 45 minutes
Servings: 4

Ingredients:

1 pound chorizo, chopped
12 ounces canned green chilies, chopped
1 yellow onion, chopped
½ teaspoon garlic powder
Salt and black pepper to the taste
1 cauliflower head, florets separated
4 eggs, whisked
2 tablespoons green onions, chopped

Directions:

1. Heat up a pan over medium heat, add chorizo and onion, stir and brown for a few minutes.
2. Add green chilies, stir, cook for a few minutes and take off heat.
3. In your food processor mix cauliflower with some salt and pepper and blend.
4. Transfer this to a bowl, add eggs, salt, pepper and garlic powder and whisk everything.
5. Add chorizo mix as well, whisk again and transfer everything to a greased baking dish.
6. Bake in the oven at 375 degrees F and bake for 40 minutes.
7. Leave casserole to cool down for a few minutes, sprinkle green onions on top, slice and serve.
Enjoy!

Nutrition: calories 350, fat 12, fiber 4, carbs 6, protein 20

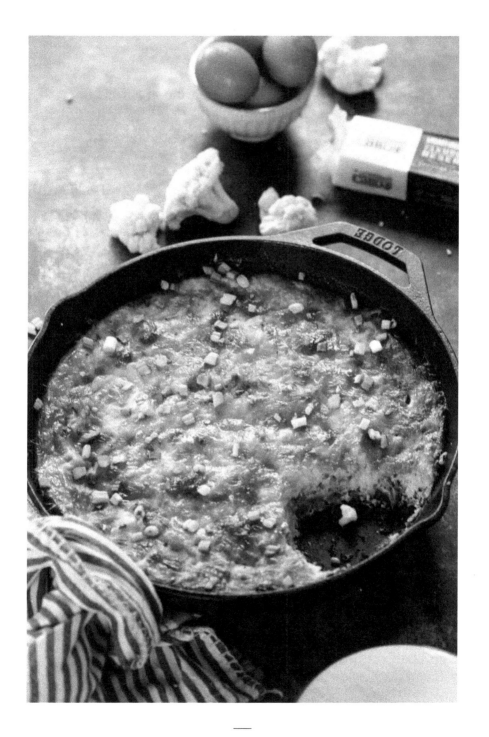

Italian Spaghetti Casserole

Try an Italian Ketogenic breakfast today!

Preparation time: 10 minutes Cooking time: 55 minutes
Servings: 4

Ingredients:

4 tablespoons ghee
1 squash, halved
Salt and black pepper to the taste
½ cup tomatoes, chopped
2 garlic cloves, minced
1 cup yellow onion, chopped
½ teaspoon Italian seasoning
3 ounces Italian salami, chopped
½ cup kalamata olives, chopped
4 eggs
A handful parsley, chopped

Directions:

1. Place squash halves on a lined baking sheet, season with salt and pepper, spread 1 tablespoon ghee over them, introduce in the oven at 400 degrees F and bake for 45 minutes.
2. Meanwhile, heat up a pan with the rest of the ghee over medium heat, add garlic, onions, salt and pepper, stir and cook for a couple of minutes.
3. Add salami and tomatoes, stir and cook for 10 minutes.
4. Add olives, stir and cook for a few minutes more.
5. Take squash halves out of the oven, scrape flesh with a fork and add over salami mix into the pan.
6. Stir, make 4 holes in the mix, crack an egg in each, season with salt and pepper, introduce pan in the oven at 400 degrees F and bake until eggs are done.
7. Sprinkle parsley on top and serve.
Enjoy!

Nutrition: calories 333, fat 23, fiber 4, carbs 12, protein 15

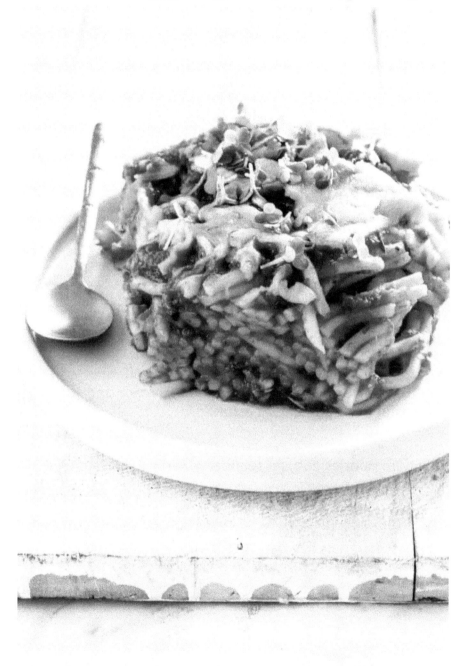

Simple Breakfast Porridge

This is just delicious!

Preparation time: 5 minutes Cooking time: 10 minutes
Servings: 1

Ingredients:

1 teaspoon cinnamon powder
A pinch of nutmeg
½ cup almonds, ground
1 teaspoon stevia
¾ cup coconut cream
A pinch of cardamom, ground
A pinch of cloves, ground

Directions:

1. Heat up a pan over medium heat, add coconut cream and heat up for a few minutes.
2. Add stevia and almonds and stir well for 5 minutes.
3. Add cloves, cardamom, nutmeg and cinnamon and stir well.
4. Transfer to a bowl and serve hot.
Enjoy!

Nutrition: calories 200, fat 12, fiber 4, carbs 8, protein 16

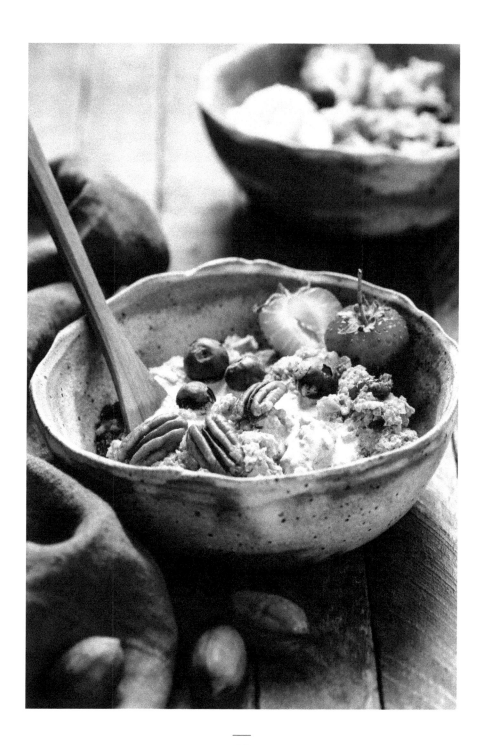

Delicious Granola

A Ketogenic breakfast granola is the best idea ever!

Preparation time: 10 minutes Cooking time: 0 minutes
Servings: 2

Ingredients:

2 tablespoons chocolate, chopped
7 strawberries, chopped
A splash of lemon juice
2 tablespoons pecans, chopped

Directions:

1. In a bowl, mix chocolate with strawberries, pecans and lemon juice.
2. Stir and serve cold.
Enjoy!

Nutrition: calories 200, fat 5, fiber 4, carbs 7, protein 8

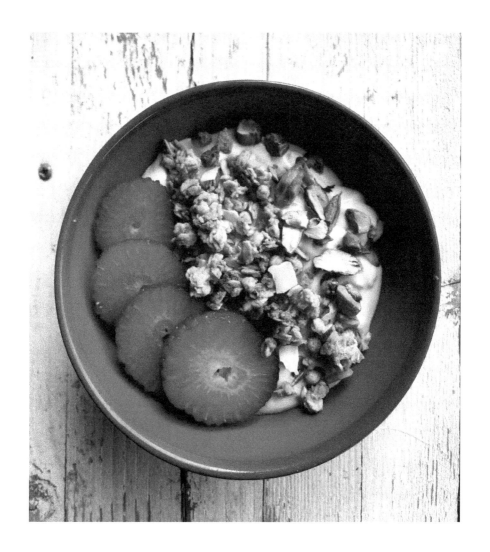

Delicious Almond Cereal

It's a great way to start your day!

Preparation time: 5 minutes Cooking time: 0 minutes.
Servings: 1

Ingredients:

2 tablespoons almonds, chopped
2 tablespoon pepitas, roasted
1/3 cup coconut milk
1 tablespoon chia seeds
1/3 cup water
A handful blueberries1 small banana, chopped

Directions:

1. In a bowl, mix chia seeds with coconut milk and leave aside for 5 minutes.
2. In your food processor, mix half of the pepitas with almonds and pulse them well.
3. Add this to chia seeds mix.
4. Also add the water and stir.
5. Top with the rest of the pepitas, banana pieces and blueberries and serve.
Enjoy!

Nutrition: calories 200, fat 3, fiber 2, carbs 5, protein 4

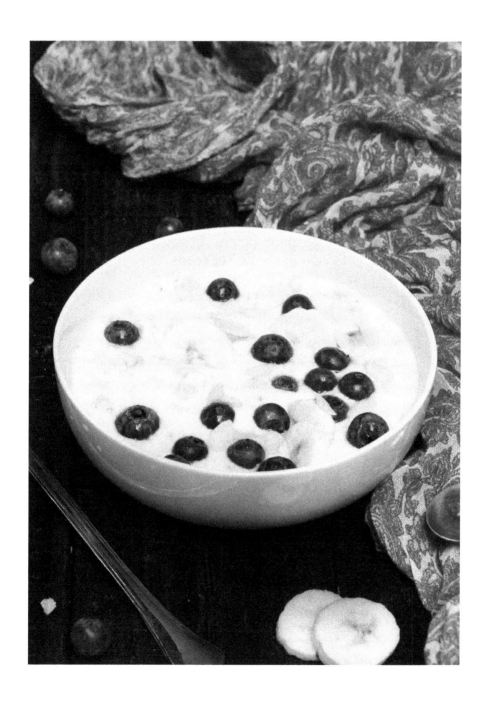

Great Breakfast Bowl

You will be surprised! It's amazing!

Preparation time: 5 minutes Cooking time: 0 minutes
Servings: 1

Ingredients:

1 teaspoon pecans, chopped
1 cup coconut milk
1 teaspoon walnuts, chopped
1 teaspoon pistachios, chopped
1 teaspoon almonds, chopped
1 teaspoon pine nuts, raw
1 teaspoon sunflower seeds, raw
1 teaspoon raw honey
1 teaspoon pepitas, raw
2 teaspoons raspberries

Directions:

1. In a bowl, mix milk with honey and stir.
2. Add pecans, walnuts, almonds, pistachios, sunflower seeds, pine nuts and pepitas.
3. Stir, top with raspberries and serve.
Enjoy!

Nutrition: calories 100, fat 2, fiber 4, carbs 5, protein 6

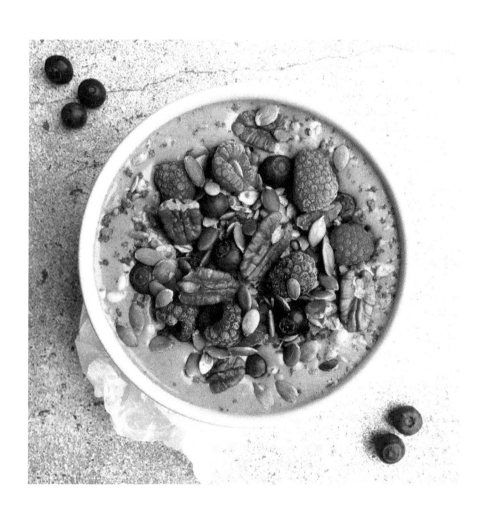

Delightful Breakfast Bread

This is a Ketogenic breakfast idea you should try soon!

Preparation time: 10 minutes Cooking time: 3 minutes
Servings: 4

Ingredients:

½ teaspoon baking powder
1/3 cup almond flour
1 egg, whisked
A pinch of salt
2 and ½ tablespoons coconut oil

Directions:

1. Grease a mug with some of the oil.
2. In a bowl, mix the egg with flour, salt, oil and baking powder and stir.
3. Pour this into the mug and cook in your microwave for 3 minutes at a High temperature.
4. Leave the bread to cool down a bit, take out of the mug, slice and serve with a glass of almond milk for breakfast.
Enjoy!

Nutrition: calories 132, fat 12, fiber 1, carbs 3, protein 4

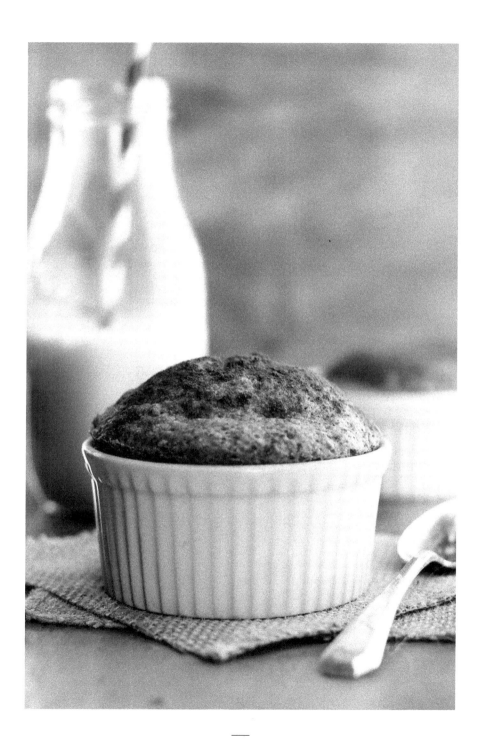

Breakfast Muffins

These will really make your day much easier!

Preparation time: 10 minutes Cooking time: 30 minutes
Servings: 4

Ingredients:

½ cup almond milk
6 eggs
1 tablespoon coconut oil
Salt and black pepper to the taste
¼ cup kale, chopped
8 prosciutto slices
¼ cup chives, chopped

Directions:

1. In a bowl, mix eggs with salt, pepper, milk, chives and kale and stir well.
2. Grease a muffin tray with melted coconut oil, line with prosciutto slices, pour eggs mix, introduce in the oven and bake at 350 degrees F for 30 minutes.
3. Transfer muffins to a platter and serve for breakfast. Enjoy!

Nutrition: calories 140, fat 3, fiber 1, carbs 3, protein 10

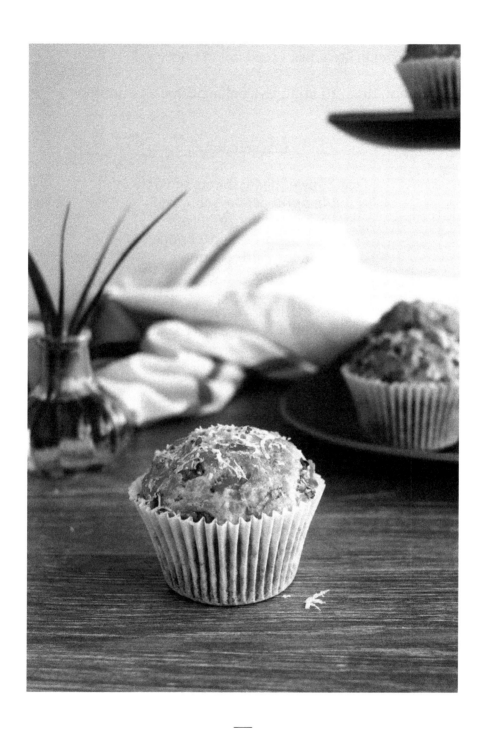

Special Breakfast Bread

It's a Ketogenic breakfast bread full of nutrients!

Preparation time: 10 minutes Cooking time: 25 minutes
Servings: 7

Ingredients:

1 cauliflower head, florets separated
A handful parsley, chopped
1 cup spinach, torn
1 small yellow onion, chopped
1 tablespoon coconut oil
½ cup pecans, ground
3 eggs
2 garlic cloves, minced
Salt and black pepper to the taste

Directions:

1. In your food processor, mix cauliflower florets with some salt and pepper and pulse well.
2. Heat up a pan with the oil over medium heat, add cauliflower, onion, garlic some salt and pepper, stir and cook for 10 minutes.
3. In a bowl, mix eggs with salt, pepper, parsley, spinach and nuts and stir.
4. Add cauliflower mix and stir well again.
5. Spread this into 7 rounds on a baking sheet, heat up the oven to 350 degrees F and bake for 15 minutes.
6. Serve these tasty breads for breakfast.
Enjoy!

Nutrition: calories 140, fat 3, fiber 3, carbs 4, protein 8

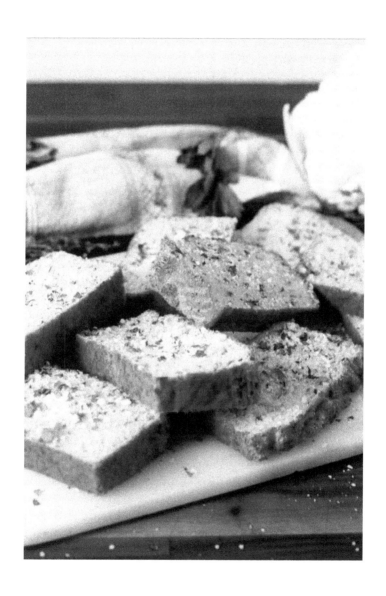

Breakfast Sandwich

It's a tasty Ketogenic breakfast sandwich! Try it soon!

Preparation time: 10 minutes Cooking time: 10 minutes
Servings: 1

Ingredients:

2 eggs
Salt and black pepper to the taste
2 tablespoons ghee
¼ pound pork sausage meat, minced
¼ cup water
1 tablespoon guacamole

Directions:

1. In a bowl, mix minced sausage meat with salt and pepper to the taste and stir well.
2. Shape a patty from this mix and place on a working surface.
3. Heat up a pan with 1 tablespoon ghee over medium heat, add sausage patty, fry for 3 minutes on each side and transfer to a plate.
4. Crack an egg in 2 bowls and whisk them a bit with some salt and pepper.
5. Heat up a pan with the rest of the ghee over medium high heat, place 2 biscuit cutters which you've greased with some ghee before in the pan and pour an egg in each.
6. Add the water to the pan, reduce heat, cover pan and cook eggs for 3 minutes.
7. Transfer these egg "buns" to paper towels and drain grease.
8. Place sausage patty on one egg "bun" spread guacamole over it and top with the other egg "bun".
Enjoy!

Nutrition: calories 200, fat 4, fiber 6, carbs 5, protein 10

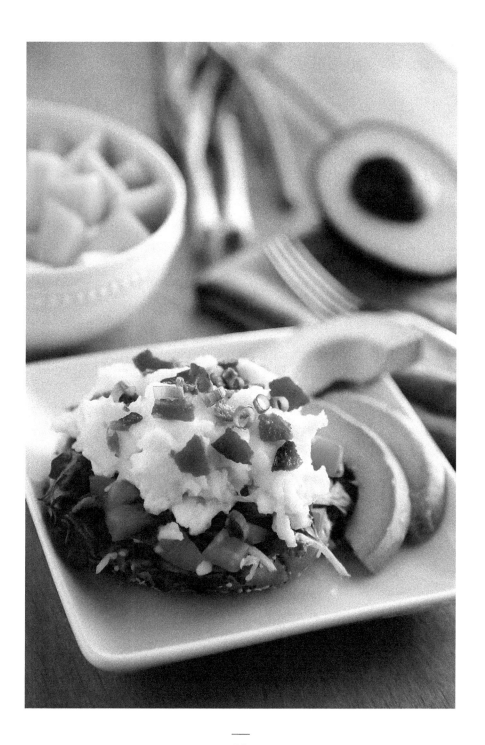

Delicious Chicken Breakfast Muffins

It's a savory Ketogenic breakfast you can try today!

Preparation time: 10 minutes Cooking time: 1 hour Servings: 3

Ingredients:

¾ pound chicken breast, boneless
Salt and black pepper to the taste
½ teaspoon garlic powder
3 tablespoons hot sauce mixed with 3 tablespoons melted
coconut oil
6 eggs
2 tablespoons green onions, chopped

Directions:

1. Season chicken breast with salt, pepper and garlic powder, place on a lined baking sheet and bake in the oven at 425 degrees F for 25 minutes.
2. Transfer chicken breast to a bowl, shred with a fork and mix with half of the hot sauce and melted coconut oil.
3. Toss to coat and leave aside for now.
4. In a bowl, mix eggs with salt, pepper, green onions and the rest of the hot sauce mixed with oil and whisk very well.
5. Divide this mix into a muffin tray, top each with shredded chicken, introduce in the oven at 350 degrees F and bake for 30 minutes.
6. Serve your muffins hot.
Enjoy!

Nutrition: calories 140, fat 8, fiber 1, carbs 2, protein 13

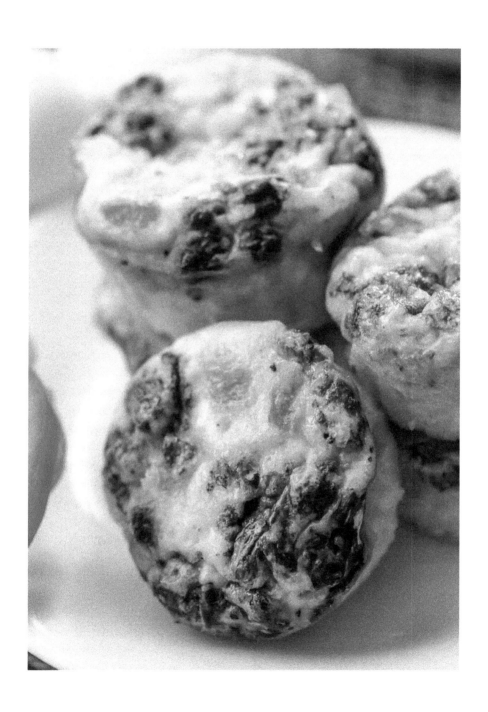

Delicious Herbed Biscuits

Try this healthy keto breakfast biscuits really soon! They are so delicious!

Preparation time: 10 minutes Cooking time: 15 minutes
Servings: 6

Ingredients:

6 tablespoons coconut oil
6 tablespoons coconut flour
2 garlic cloves, minced
¼ cup yellow onion, minced
2 eggs
Salt and black pepper to the taste
1 tablespoons parsley, chopped
2 tablespoons coconut milk
½ teaspoon apple cider vinegar
¼ teaspoon baking soda

Directions:

1. In a bowl, mix coconut flour with eggs, oil, garlic, onion, coconut milk, parsley, salt and pepper and stir well.
2. In a bowl, mix vinegar with baking soda, stir well and add to the batter.
3. Drop spoonful of this batter on lined baking sheets and shape circles.
4. Introduce in the oven at 350 degrees F and bake for 15 minutes.
5. Serve these biscuits for breakfast.
Enjoy!

Nutrition: calories 140, fat 6, fiber 2, carbs 10, protein 12

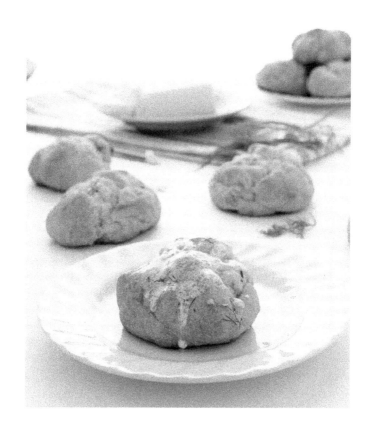